DIABETIC COOKBOOK

FOR BEGINNERS

45+ Mouth-watering, Easy-to-cook, Low-carb Diabetic Recipes to Fulfill Your Cravings of Sweets, Maintaining your Health, and Recover From Diabetes in this Diabetic Dessert Cookbook Beginners can Follow.

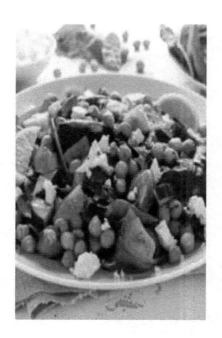

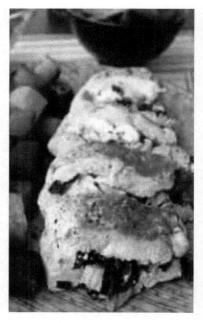

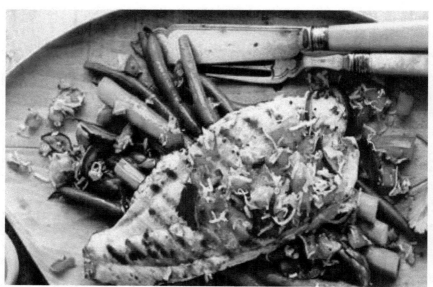

Table of Contents

INTRODUCTION

Diabetes can be all around made do with good dieting, joined with standard actual work and weight management. If you have diabetes, it is suggested that you follow a good dieting plan dependent on a lot of vegetables and vegetables (like chickpeas, lentils, low-salt prepared beans and kidney beans). Incorporate some high-fiber sugar food varieties, for example, wholegrain breads and grains and organic product, just as some lean protein sources and diminished fat dairy items. Diminish your admission of soaked (undesirable) fat and added sugars, and pick food varieties low in salt. Decreasing the serving size of your dinners can likewise assist you with keeping a sound body weight and takes into account better blood glucose the executives. It is suggested that you see a dietitian who can work with you to build up a good dieting plan that is perfect for you.

Diabetic meals recipes

30+ recipes

1. Sheet Pan Seafood Bake

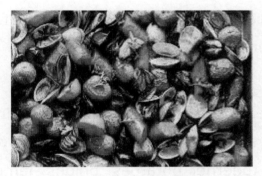

Active: 15 mins | Total: 40 mins | Yield: Serves 4 (serving size: about 5 1/3 oz.)

Ingredients

- 12 ounces baby red potatoes
- 2 small yellow onions, cut into 1-in. wedges
- 2 lemons, halved crosswise
- 3 tablespoons olive oil
- 1 ½ teaspoons Cajun seafood boil seasoning (such as Slap Ya Mama Cajun Seafood Boil)
- 2 pounds littleneck clams in shells, scrubbed

- 12 ounces smoked andouille sausage, cut into 2-in. pieces
- 1 pound fresh mussels in shells, scrubbed
- ½ cup dry white wine
- ¼ cup salted butter, melted
- 1 tablespoon hot sauce (such as Crystal)
- 1 ½ teaspoons Worcestershire sauce
- 2 tablespoons chopped fresh flat-leaf parsley
- Lemon wedges, for serving

Direction

1. Preheat oven to 450°F with 1 rack in top third of oven and 1 rack in bottom third of oven. Toss together potatoes, onions, lemon halves, oil, and seafood boils seasoning on an aluminum-foil-lined rimmed baking sheet. Spread in an even layer, and roast in preheated oven on bottom rack until potatoes are just tender, about 25 minutes.

2. Spread clams on a second foil-lined rimmed baking sheet. Bake at 450°F on top rack just until clams begin to open, 8 to 10 minutes.

3. When potatoes have roasted 25 minutes and clams have opened, spread andouille evenly on baking sheet with potatoes, and spread

mussels evenly over clams. Pour wine over clam mixture. Bake until mussels have opened, about 8 minutes.

4. Stir together butter, hot sauce, and Worcestershire sauce. Spread potato mixture evenly over clams and mussels on baking sheet. Drizzle evenly with butter sauce, and sprinkle evenly with parsley. Garnish with lemon wedges, and serve immediately.

2. Beef Lettuce Cups with Carrots

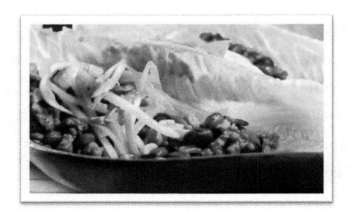

SERVINGS 4 | PREP TIME 40 min | COOK TIME 5 min | DURATION 45 min

Ingredients

- 1/4 cup rice vinegar
- 1 tbsp. plus 1/2 tsp. raw honey, divided
- 1/8 tsp. sea salt
- 1 carrot, peeled and cut into matchsticks (1/ cup)
- 1 daikon radish, cut into matchsticks (1/cup) (TIP: If you can't find daikon radish, regular radish works well here too.)
- 1 tsp. sesame oil
- 10 oz. lean ground beef
- 1/2 cup finely chopped red onion

- 3 cloves garlic, minced
- 1 tbsp. peeled and minced fresh ginger
- 1 1/3 cups BPA-free canned unsalted black beans, drained and rinsed
- 1 tbsp. reduced-sodium soy sauce
- 12 romaine lettuce leaves
- 2 tbsp. chopped roasted unsalted peanuts
- 2 tbsp. thinly sliced scallions

Preparation

1. Firstly In a medium bowl, whisk together vinegar, 1 tbsp. honey and salt. Add carrot and radish; toss to coat. Cover and transfer to refrigerator to marinate until tender and chilled, at least 2 hours or overnight.

2. Heat a large nonstick skillet on medium and brush with oil. Then Add beef and sauté until no longer pink, about 5 minutes. Push beef to one side of skillet. To other side, add onion, garlic and ginger; sauté until onion softens, about 2 minutes.

3. Add beans, soy sauce and remaining 1/2 tsp. honey and stir all ingredients together; simmer for 3 minutes, stirring occasionally.

4. Drain liquid from slaw. Fill in each lettuce leaf with 1/4 cup beef-bean mixture; top it with slaw. Garnish with peanuts and scallions.

3. Sausage Stuffing casserole

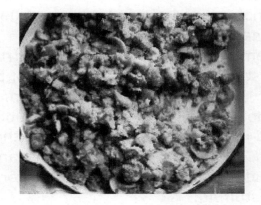

Prep/Total Time: 25 min.| Makes: 8 servings
Ingredients
- 1 pound mass pork sausage
- 1-1/4 cups chopped celery
- 1/2 cup chopped onion
- 1/2 cup cut new mushrooms
- 1 enormous garlic clove, minced
- 1-1/2 cups diminished sodium chicken stock
- 1 teaspoon scoured sage
- 1 bundle (6 ounces) stuffing blend

Directions
1. In an enormous skillet, cook the frankfurter, celery, onion and mushrooms over medium heat until meat is not, at this point pink. Add garlic; cook brief longer; channel. Mix in stock and sage.

2. Heat to the point of boiling. Mix in stuffing blend. Cover and eliminate from the heat; let represent 5 minutes. Cushion with a fork.
3. Dried spices have their place in a lot of recipes; however stuffing isn't one of them. Attempt a blend of new parsley, sage, rosemary and thyme,
4. Custom made bread garnishes will truly make your stuffing sparkle. Any portion of bread will work; top choices are nation portion, sourdough, and brioche or rye portion. Cut the bread into 1-inch solid shapes and throw them into a 300°F oven until they're dry and fresh, around 45 minutes. Get more tips for best-truly stuffing.

4.   Shrimp soup

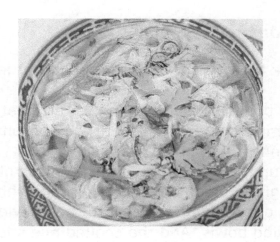

Preparation: 10 min| Cooking: 10 min| 260 calories| 2 servings

Ingredients
- 3 cups chicken stock
- 80 g rice sticks (noodles)
- 1 carrots, ground
- 2 button (white) mushrooms, daintily cut
- 9 tbsp. green cabbage, or Savoy, daintily cut
- 2 green onions/scallions, daintily cut
- 14 shrimp, medium-huge
- 1/4 tsp. gingerroot, ground
- 1 clove garlic, minced
- ½ dried stew peppers, minced
- 2 tbsp. lime juice, newly crushed
- 2 tsp. fresh cilantro [optional]
- 1 pinch salt [optional]
- Before you start

- Singular 500 ml (2 cups) serving bowls are required.

Instructions:

1. Cook the rice sticks at that point put in a safe spot.
2. In a pot of salted bubbling water, heat up the shrimp around 3 min, until they become pink. Channel and put in a safe spot.
3. Set up the vegetables. Mesh the carrots, cut the green onions, cabbage, and mushrooms. Part out the vegetables into the individual serving bowls. Add the cooked rice sticks.
4. Heat the stock in a pot. Add the ground ginger, minced garlic and stew pepper. Cook 2 min. Add the cooked shrimp and cook an extra 3-4 min. Change the flavoring.
5. Empty the hot stock into the serving bowls. Add the lime juice, decorate with entire cilantro leaves, and serve.

5.   Fish Cakes Recipe

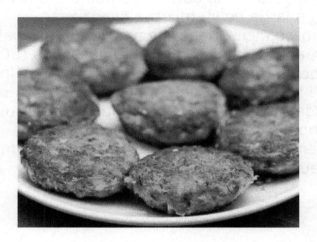

Prep time: 15 minutes | Cooking time: 20 minutes | Yield: 4 servings

INGREDIENTS:

- For salmon fish cakes -
- 3 tins of salmon (approx. 450 g), drained and flaked (or use salmon fillet and cook them first)
- 2 tablespoons of fresh dill (6 g), finely chopped
- 3 medium eggs, beaten
- 1/4 cup of coconut flour (28 g)
- 1/4 cup of grated coconut (20 g)
- 1/4 cup of coconut oil (60 ml)
- Salt and pepper , to taste

For preparing fish cakes -

- 2 tablespoons of coconut oil (30 ml)
- For creamy dill sauce -
- 1/4 cup of mayonnaise (60 ml)
- 1/4 cup of coconut milk (60 ml) (can at room temperature)
- 2 cloves of garlic (6 g), finely chopped or diced
- 2 teaspoons of fresh dill (2 g), chopped

- Salt and pepper , to taste

DIRECTIONS:

1. Beat in a small bowl to combine the dill sauce
2. In a large bowl, mix the fishcake thoroughly. Shape the mixture into 8 patties.
3. In a large skillet, melt 2 tablespoons (30 ml) of coconut oil. Carefully place the patties in the oil in batches. Cook until golden brown on one side then flips and cook until golden brown, about 3 to 4 minutes per side.
4. Serve the salmon patties with the creamy dill sauce.

6. Salmon with salad and eggs

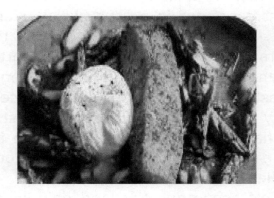

Total: 45 mins | Servings: 4

Ingredients

- 1 tablespoon coriander seeds
- 1 teaspoon lemon zing
- ¾ teaspoon fine ocean salt, separated
- ½ teaspoon squashed red pepper
- 1 pound wild salmon , skin-on, cut into 4 parts
- 1 pound asparagus, managed
- 2 tablespoons extra-virgin olive oil
- 1 tablespoon lemon juice
- 1 tablespoon chopped new mint
- 1 tablespoon chopped new tarragon
- ¼ teaspoon ground pepper, in addition to additional for embellish
- 8 cups water
- 1 tablespoon white vinegar
- 4 huge eggs

Directions:

1. Position a rack in upper third of oven; preheat grill to high. Coat a rimmed preparing sheet with cooking splash.
2. Toast coriander in a little skillet over medium heat, shaking the pan much of the time, until fragrant, around 3 minutes. Heartbeat the coriander, lemon zing, 1/2 teaspoon salt and squashed red pepper in a zest processor until finely ground. Coat the salmon substance with the flavor combination (around 1/2 teaspoons for each bit) and spot the salmon on the readied preparing sheet.
3. Cut off asparagus tips and daintily cut stalks on the inclining. Throw the tips and cuts with oil, lemon juice, mint, tarragon, pepper and the remaining 1/4 teaspoon salt. Let stand while you cook the salmon and eggs.
4. Heat water and vinegar to the point of boiling in a huge saucepan.
5. In the interim, sear the salmon until just cooked through, 3 to 6 minutes, contingent upon thickness Tent with foil to keep warm.
6. Decrease the bubbling water to an exposed stew. Delicately mix in a circle so the water is whirling around the pot. Break eggs, each in turn, into the water. Cook until the whites are set yet the yolks are as yet runny, 3 to 4 minutes.
7. To serve, partition the asparagus serving of mixed greens and salmon among 4 plates. Make a home in every serving of mixed greens and top with a poached egg.

7.   Parsley Roast Tilapia

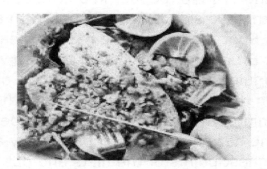

Active: 20 mins | Total: 30 mins| Servings: 4 (4 x 11)

Ingredients
- 2 tablespoons olive oil, partitioned
- 4 (5 ounce) tilapia filets (new or frozen, defrosted)
- ⅓ cup finely chopped hazelnuts
- ¼ cup finely chopped new parsley
- 1 little shallot, minced
- 2 teaspoons lemon zing
- ⅛ teaspoon salt in addition to 1/4 teaspoon, partitioned
- ¼ teaspoon ground pepper, partitioned
- 1 ½ tablespoons lemon juice

Directions:
1. Preheat oven to 450 degrees F. Line a huge rimmed preparing sheet with foil; brush with 1 Tbsp. oil. Carry fish to room temperature by allowing it to remain on the counter for 15 minutes.

2. In the mean time, mix together hazelnuts, parsley, shallot, lemon zing, 1 tsp. oil, 1/8 tsp. salt, and 1/8 tsp. pepper in a little bowl.
3. Wipe the two sides of the fish off with a paper towel. Spot the fish on the readied heating sheet. Brush the two sides of the fish with lemon juice and the remaining 2 tsp. oil. Season the two sides equitably with the remaining 1/4 tsp. salt and 1/8 tsp. pepper. Gap the hazelnut combination equally among the highest points of the filets and pat tenderly to follow.
4. Broil the fish until it is obscure, firm, and simply starting to piece, 7 to 10 minutes. Serve right away.

8.   Lemon Garlic Salmon with Asparagus

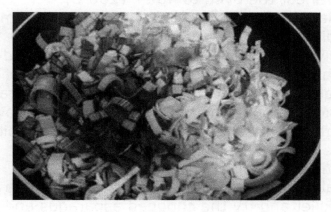

Prep time: 10 minutes | Cooking time: 20 minutes | Yield: 2 servings

INGREDIENTS:

- For the ghee salmon with lemon garlic:
- 2 salmon fillets (skin on), fresh or frozen (340 g), thaw if frozen
- 1 tablespoon (15 ml) ghee (use avocado oil for AIP)
- 4 cloves of garlic (12 g), chopped
- 2 teaspoons (10 ml) lemon juice
- Salt to taste
- Lemon slices to serve

For the leek, asparagus and ginger roast:

- 10 asparagus (160 g), chopped into small pieces
- 1 leek (90 g), chopped into small pieces
- 2 teaspoons (4 g) ginger powder (or use finely chopped fresh ginger if you have it available)
- Avocado oil or olive oil to fry with
- 1 tablespoon of lemon juice

- Salt to taste

DIRECTIONS:
1. Preheat the oven to 400 F (200 C).
2. Place each salmon fillet on a piece of aluminum foil or baking paper.
3. Divide the ghee, lemon juice and chopped garlic over the two fillets - place on top of the salmon. Sprinkle with some salt. Then wrap the salmon in the foil and place it in the oven.
4. After 10 minutes in the oven, open the foil and bake for another 10 minutes.
5. While the salmon is cooking, put 1-2 tablespoons of avocado oil or olive oil in a skillet and fry the chopped asparagus and leeks over high heat. Bake for 10 minutes and then add the ginger powder, lemon juice and salt to taste. Bake for 1 minute more.
6. Serve by dividing the sauté over 2 plates and placing a salmon fillet on each plate.

9. Caesar Salad Recipe

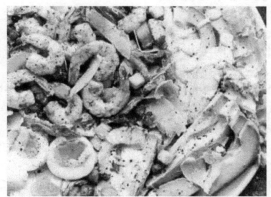

Prep Time: 15 minutes | Cooking Time: 10 minutes | Yield: 4 servings

INGREDIENTS:
For the shrimp:
- 1 pound shrimp (shell removed)
- 2 tablespoons of olive oil
- 1 tablespoon of lemon juice
- 3 tablespoons of garlic powder
- 1 tablespoon of onion powder
- Salt and pepper

For the salad:
- 1 head of romaine lettuce, chopped
- 1 cucumber, cut into cubes
- For the dressing:
- 1 teaspoon of Dijon mustard
- 1/4 cup Paleo-mayonnaise (you can buy them or make them yourself)
- 1 tablespoon of fresh lemon juice
- 2 teaspoons of garlic powder
- Salt and pepper

For garnish:
- 1 tablespoon of parsley, chopped - for garnish

- 1 tablespoon sliced almonds - for garnish

DIRECTIONS:

1. Preheat the oven to 400F.
2. Mix the shrimps, olive oil, lemon juice, garlic, and onion powder, salt and pepper together. Place the shrimp on the baking tray and roast for 10 minutes.
3. To make the salad dressing, mix together the mayo, mustard, lemon juice, garlic powder, salt and pepper.
4. Toss the dressing with the chopped lettuce, chopped cucumber, and roasted shrimp. Garnish with the chopped parsley and sliced almonds.

10. Vegan bowl

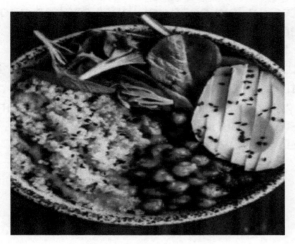

INGREDIENTS:
- Spicy marinated tofu
- Firm tofu cut into 1-inch cubes
- Buddha bowl
- Mushrooms, sliced
- Cauliflower, cut into florets
- Broccoli, cut into small florets
- Baby bok choy

DIRECTIONS:
1. Spicy marinated tofu
2. Mixing
3. Well until all of the tofu is evenly coated.
4. Line a large baking dish with parchment paper
5. And divide the tofu into a single layer.
6. Buddha bowl
7. Set the mushrooms aside.
8. Toss in the cauliflower rice
9. The pan along with the chopped parsley and cook until soft, approx. For 10 minutes.
10. Microwave on high heat, approx. 5 minutes.
11. Add a splash of boiling water

12. To a medium skillet and place the bok choy in it, cut side down. Cook for 3-5
13. Minutes on low heat until just cooked and tender.
14. Place the
15. Broccoli and bok choy on the other side. Top with fried mushrooms and
16. Crispy marinated tofu. Garnish with sesame seeds and chili, if desired. Salt and
17. Pepper to taste.

11. Miso Soup Recipe

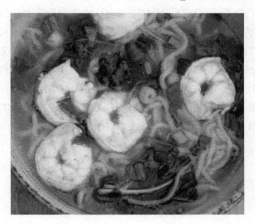

Prep Time: 10 minutes | Cooking Time: 0 minutes | Yield: 2 servings

INGREDIENTS:
- 2 (85 g) cartons of shirataki noodles, drained
- cups of chicken broth (600 ml) and bone broth
- 1 tablespoon of tahini sauce (15 ml)
- 1 tablespoon of gluten - free tamari sauce or coconut aminos (15 ml)
- 1/2-pound shrimp (225 g), peeled
- 1 teaspoon of sesame oil (5 ml)
- 2 tablespoons of lemon juice (30 ml)
- 2 green onions (10 g), sliced diagonally
- 1 cup of spinach (30 g), thinly sliced
- Pinch of hot sauce (optional)

DIRECTIONS:
1. Rinse the shirataki noodles well, following the package *DIRECTIONS:* to remove the odor. It also helps to boil it up a bit and then rinse it off again. Drain and set aside.

2. Heat the stock and add the tahini sauce and tamari sauce. Once steamed, add the shrimp, sesame oil, and lemon juice and keep the heat until you're sure the shrimp are cooked.
3. Add the drained noodles along with the green onions and thinly sliced spinach to the stock and heat through.
4. Divide between 2 bowls and serve immediately with a splash of hot sauce.

12. Vegan Pho Recipe

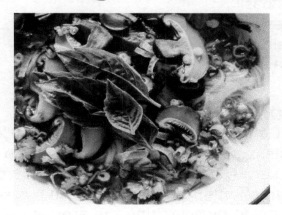

Prep time: 30 min | Cook time: 5 min |Servings: 2

INGREDIENTS
- Vegetarian Pho Stock
- 2.5 onions, divided
- 2 creeps of ginger, cut
- 2 pieces cinnamon (4" each)
- 5 star anise
- 1 tablespoon fennel seeds
- 1 teaspoon coriander seeds
- 1 teaspoon cardamom units
- 1/2 teaspoon cloves (10)
- 25 dried shiitake mushrooms
- 1 lb. daikon, stripped and cut into 1 inch pieces
- Salt and sugar, to taste
- To Serve
- Pho noodles
- Meagerly cut onion
- Different sorts of tofu
- Lord shellfish mushrooms, sautéed
- Wood ear mushrooms

- Cut green onions and cilantro
- Thai basil
- Limes
- Hoisin sauce
- Sriracha

DIRECTIONS:

1. Heat a huge pot of water to the point of boiling – this is so the Instant Pot gets up to pressure quicker. Don't hesitate to avoid this progression in case you're not in a rush.
2. Get going by scorching the aromatics. Spot the onion, ginger, cinnamon stick, star anise, fennel seeds, coriander seeds, cardamom units, and cloves on a rimmed preparing sheet and blow light until fragrant. On the other hand, roast the onions and ginger on an open air barbecue, over a gas range, or in an oven and toast the flavors in a dry skillet on low heat until they are sweet-smelling, around 2-3 minutes. Tie the flavors up in cheesecloth or huge tea/zest sack for simple expulsion from your soup.
3. Add the flavors to the Instant Pot along the shiitakes, ginger, and daikon. Add the heated water to the addition, up to the 4 quart line. Put the cover on; set the strain too high for 45 minutes. Fast delivery when it's set, at that point cautiously eliminates the entirety of the mushrooms and aromatics. On the off chance that you have the opportunity, regular delivery is the better alternative as it'll keep in a greater amount of the flavors.

4. Season the pho stock with salt and sugar, being certain to prepare forcefully in light of the fact that the stock should enhance the noodles and garnishes also. We do 1-2 teaspoons of salt and 2 tablespoons of sugar for each quart of fluid after the solids are stressed out.
5. For fixings, you can keep the mushrooms from the stock, just let them cool somewhat, at that point trim the stems and cut. We likewise added two sorts of tofu: medium firm and seared, just as some sautéed kind clam mushrooms and wood ear mushrooms.
6. To serve: Prepare the noodles as indicated by the bundle, strain and gap equitably into enormous, profound dishes. Add a liberal measure of mushrooms and tofu. Top with a liberal measure of stock. Present with limes, Thai basil, daintily cut onions and cilantro and bean stews. Have little plunging plates of sriracha and hoisin sauces for every individual. Enjoy right away!

13. Collard Greens

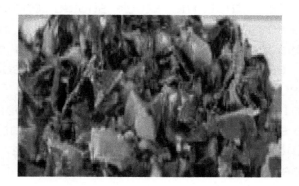

Prep time: 30 min| Servings: 5| Ingredients

INGREDIENTS:
- 1 tablespoon olive oil
- 1 little white onion finely diced
- 3 cloves garlic minced
- 3 cups chicken stock
- 1 teaspoon red pepper drops
- 1 large smoked turkey leg completely cooked
- 32 oz. collard greens altogether washed and cut into strips.
- Salt and pepper
- Hot sauce

Directions
1. In a large profound skillet or pot, heat olive oil on medium heat.
2. Include onions and cook until delicate.
3. Mix in garlic and cook until fragrant.
4. Add chicken stock, red pepper pieces and smoked turkey.
5. Heat to the point of boiling and diminish heat.

6. Cover and bubble daintily for around 20-30 minutes.
7. Eliminate turkey leg and let cool.
8. Eliminate meat from bone and cut into scaled down pieces.
9. Return meat and skin back to the pot.
10. Stew for 10 minutes.
11. Add collard greens to pot, pushing them down if necessary.
12. At the point when greens start to shrink down, cover and stew for as long as an hour or until your ideal surface is reached, mixing sometimes.
13. Add salt and pepper whenever wanted.
14. Plate the greens and pour on a couple of drops of hot sauce.

14. Steak Marinade

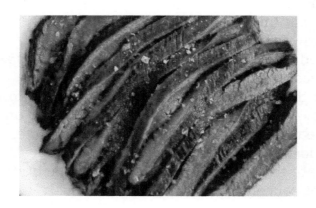

PREP TIME: 10 mins | COOK TIME: 14 mins | TOTAL TIME: 24 mins | SERVINGS: 4 servings

INGREDIENTS:
- (1/2-to 2-pound) flank steak
- 1/4 cup low sodium soy sauce
- 1/4 cup balsamic vinegar
- 1/2 cup vegetable oil
- 3 Tablespoons nectar
- 4 cloves garlic, minced
- 2 Tablespoons minced new ginger
- 3 scallions, meagerly cut
- Hardware:
- gallon size sealable plastic pack

INSTRUCTIONS:

1. Spot the plastic pack in a huge bowl and afterward add the soy sauce, balsamic vinegar, oil and nectar to the sack. Speed in the garlic, ginger and scallions. Add the steak to the sack, flipping it to cover it in the marinade, and afterward seal the plastic pack.
2. Spot the steak in the cooler and marinate it short-term, or for at least 10 hours.
3. At the point when prepared to cook, eliminate the steak from the cooler and preheat your cooking surface (flame broil or burner barbecue dish). Eliminate the steak from the marinade, dispose of the extra fluid, and singe the steak on each side until it's cooked to your ideal level of doneness. Allow the steak to rest for 5 minutes and afterward cut it contrary to what would be expected and serve.

15. Green detox salad

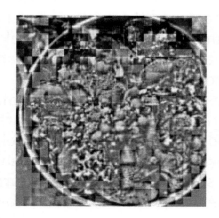

Prep time 30 minutes |Cook time 30 minutes | Total time 1 hour| Servings 4 servings| Calories 348 kcal

INGREDIENTS

- LEMON TAHINI DRESSING
- 2 tablespoons tahini sesame seed paste
- 2 tablespoons olive oil
- 1 teaspoon low sodium soy sauce or tamari
- juice + zing from 1 lemon utilize just 50% of the zing
- 2 cloves garlic ground
- 2 teaspoons new ginger ground
- salt + pepper to taste
- Serving of mixed greens
- 2 cups cooked chickpeas
- 1 cup unsweetened chipped coconut
- 2 tablespoon low sodium soy sauce or tamari
- 2 tablespoons sesame oil
- 1/4 teaspoon cayenne pepper
- 4 cups Tuscan kale generally torn
- 2 cups new broccoli florets

- 1/4 head purple cabbage shredded
- 1/2 cup new parsley + cilantro generally chopped
- hemp seeds + chia seeds for garnish
- 2 red grapefruits divided
- 2 ready however firm avocados cut or chopped
- Vegetarian PARMESAN
- 1/2 cup crude pine nuts
- 2 teaspoons crude sesame seeds
- 1 tablespoon wholesome yeast
- salt to taste

GUIDELINES
1. LEMON TAHINI DRESSING
2. Add every one of the ingredients to a bowl and speed until consolidated. Taste and change salt + pepper however you would prefer. On the other hand you can add the ingredients to a blender or food processor and mix until smooth. The dressing can be made seven days ahead of time and put away in the ice chest until prepared to utilize.
3. Plate of mixed greens
4. Preheat the oven to 425 degrees F.
5. Spread the chickpeas out on a towel and dry them totally. Add the chickpeas and coconut to a preparing sheet and throw with the soy sauce, sesame oil and cayenne pepper. Throw well to uniformly cover. Broil for 20 minutes and afterward mix the chickpeas around and cook an additional 10 minutes or until the chickpeas are browned and the coconut is dim brown. Eliminate from the oven. Save any extras for eating on later!

6. Add the kale to a huge bowl and sprinkle with 1 teaspoon olive oil and a major touch of salt. Using your hands, knead the kale for 2-3 minutes until the kale is all around covered and has somewhat relaxed. To the bowl add the broccoli, cabbage, parsley, and cilantro. Throw well. Add the dressing and keep on throwing until every one of the veggies are covered. Add the grapefruit portions and avocado. Tenderly throw to consolidate. Now, you can cover and store the plate of mixed greens in the ice chest for as long as 24 hours or proceed with the formula.
7. Gap the serving of mixed greens into bowls. Top with the crunchy coconut chickpeas and the vegetarian parmesan cheddar (formula underneath) and a sprinkle of chia + hemp seeds. EAT!!
8. Vegetarian PARMESAN
9. In a food processor or blender, consolidate the pine nuts, sesame seeds, wholesome yeast and a touch of salt. Processor until you has fine scraps that look like parmesan cheddar. Taste and season with more salt whenever wanted. The veggie lover parmesan can be made seven days ahead of time and put away in the cooler until prepared to utilize.

16. Rice Noodle Soup

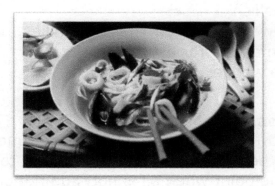

Yield 4 servings| time 1 hour

INGREDIENTS

- 2 teaspoons crude nut oil or sesame oil
- 1 huge onion, in thick cuts
- 1 3-inch piece ginger, stripped and daintily cut
- ½ cup daintily cut lemon grass
- 1 2-inch piece cinnamon stick
- 2 star anise
- 4 cloves
- ½ teaspoon coriander seeds, squashed
- ½ teaspoon fennel seeds, squashed
- 4 little dry red chilies
- ⅛ teaspoon turmeric
- 2 teaspoons sugar
- 1 tablespoon soy sauce
- 2 teaspoons Asian fish sauce
- 8 cups fish stock or chicken stock
- Salt and pepper
- 8 ounces dainty rice noodles (vermicelli)
- 2 pounds mussels, scoured
- 1 pound squid, cut 1/2-inch thick

- ½ cup generally chopped cilantro, for embellish
- ¼ cup chopped scallions, for embellish
- Leaves from 1 little bundle Thai basil, for embellish
- 6 new green or red Thai bird chilies, fragmented, for decorate
- Lime wedges, for decorate

Instructions:
1. Spot a weighty lined soup pot over medium-high heat. Add the nut oil, and twirl to cover. At the point when oil is hot, add the onion and cook for 5 minutes, blending, until relaxed and delicately browned. Add all the aromatics (ginger, lemon grass, cinnamon, star anise, cloves, coriander, fennel, dry chilies and turmeric) and mix to circulate. Add the sugar and let everything fry delicately, until sugar starts to caramelize, around 2 minutes. Add the soy sauce, fish sauce and stock. Heat to the point of boiling, at that point decrease heat to a delicate stew. Cook for 30 minutes. Strain, disposing of solids. Season to taste with the salt and a liberal measure of pepper. (May be ready a few hours ahead.)
2. Drench the rice noodles: Put the rice vermicelli in an enormous bowl. Cover with bubbling water. Mix noodles as they mollify. Drench for around 20 minutes until delicate. Cool in a colander under running water and channel. Save at room temperature.
3. To serve, carry soup to a lively stew. Add the mussels and put on the cover. Cook 2 minutes, until mussels have opened. Add the squid, mix

to join and cook 30 seconds more. Mood killer heat.

4. Separation rice noodles among 4 enormous soup bowls. Spoon soup into bowls. Sprinkle with the cilantro, scallions and Thai basil. Pass the new chilies and lime wedges independently.

17. Broccoli Rabe

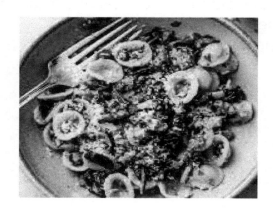

Total: 30 mins | Servings: 6 (6 trays makes 36 person serving)

Ingredients

- 2 teaspoons salt
- 12 ounces orecchiette pasta (around 3 1/2 cups)
- 2 pounds broccoli rabe (around 2 bundles)
- ¼ cup extra-virgin olive oil
- 3 cloves garlic, chopped
- ½ teaspoon squashed red pepper
- 8 anchovy filets, chopped
- 1 16 ounces cherry tomatoes, divided
- Newly ground Parmesan cheese (discretionary)

DIRECTION:

1. Heat 2 quarts of water to the point of boiling in a huge pot. Mix in salt, add pasta and cook as indicated by bundle guidelines until simply

delicate. Channel, holding 1/2 cup of the water.

2. Then, altogether wash broccoli rabe and trim off extreme closures. Cleave into 2-inch lengths. Leave a portion of the water sticking to the leaves and stems; this will help make a sauce.

3. Heat oil in a huge skillet over medium heat until it begins to gleam. Add garlic, squashed red pepper and anchovies, crushing the filets until they break up. Add the broccoli rabe (you may need to do this in bunches, mixing each group a little until it withers enough to add more). Cook, mixing, until practically delicate, 6 to 10 minutes. Add tomatoes and throw until they start to mollify, around 2 minutes. Add the pasta and throw to cover. On the off chance that it's excessively dry, add a tad bit of the saved pasta water. Serve quickly, embellished with Parmesan whenever wanted.

18. Salmon Curry

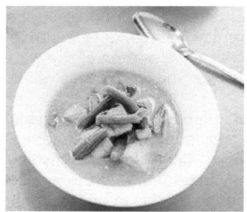

Prep Time: 10 minutes | Cooking Time: 15 minutes | Yield: 2 servings

DIRECTIONS:

- 1/2 medium onion, diced or finely chopped
- 2 cups (7 oz. or 200 g) green beans, diced
- 1.5 tablespoons (10 g) of curry powder
- 1 teaspoon (3 g) of garlic powder
- Cream the top of 1 (14-oz) can of coconut milk
- 2 cups (480 ml) of bone broth
- 1 lb. (450 g) raw salmon, diced (defrost first if frozen)
- 2 tablespoons (30 ml) of coconut oil for cooking
- Salt and pepper , to taste
- 2 tablespoons of basil (4 g), chopped, for garnish

DIRECTIONS:

1. Cook the diced onion in the coconut oil until translucent.
2. Add the green beans and cook for a few more minutes.
3. Add the stock or water and bring to the boil.

4. Add the curry powder, garlic powder and salmon.
5. Add the coconut cream and simmer until the salmon is tender (3-5 minutes).
6. Add salt and pepper to taste and serve with the chopped basil.

19. Roasted Cauliflower Broccoli

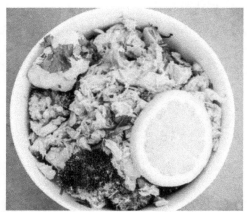

Prep time: 5 minutes | Cooking time: 20 minutes | Yield: 4 servings

INGREDIENTS:

- 1 head of cauliflower, broken into small florets
- 1 cup broccoli, broken into small florets
- Olive oil for cooking
- 1 lemon
- Salt to taste
- Four cans of tuna fish of 150 g (packed in brine, or olive oil)
- 1/4 cup fresh parsley, chopped (or use cilantro)
- For the tahini tamari pasta (omit AIP)
- 1/4 cup of tahini
- 3 tablespoons of gluten-free tamari soy sauce
- 1 tablespoon of sesame oil

DIRECTIONS:

1. Preheat the oven to 400 F (205 C).
2. Place the cauliflower and broccoli florets on a baking tray and drizzle with olive oil. Sprinkle salt and squeeze the juice of 1/4 lemon over the vegetables. Rub the mixture into the vegetables with your hands and spread them on the baking tray.
3. Place in the oven and cook for 20 minutes until the florets are tender and brown on the edges.
4. Let the vegetables cool for a few minutes, then put them in a large bowl and mix with the chopped parsley, 1 tablespoon olive oil, 1/4 lemon juice and extra salt to taste.
5. Mix all the of the pasta well to make the tahini tamari paste.
6. To serve, put the roasted vegetables in a small bowl and cover with a can of tuna. Add some tahini tamari sauce and enjoy.
7. This recipe is enough for 4 people or you can keep the leftover pasta and roasted vegetables in the fridge for future meals.

20. Sheet pan Parmesan Chicken

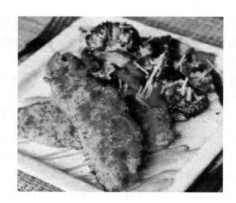

Prep: 20 min. Bake: 20 min.| Makes: 4 servings
Ingredients
- 4 boneless skinless chicken bosom parts (6 ounces each)
- 3 teaspoons olive oil, separated
- 1 teaspoon dried rosemary, squashed
- 1/2 teaspoon dried thyme
- 1/2 teaspoon pepper
- 2 jars (14 ounces each) water-stuffed artichoke hearts, depleted and quartered
- 1 medium onion, coarsely chopped
- 1/2 cup white wine or decreased sodium chicken stock
- 2 garlic cloves, chopped
- 1/4 cup shredded Parmesan cheddar
- 1 lemon, cut into 8 cuts
- 2 green onions, daintily cut

Directions
1. Preheat oven to 375°. Spot chicken in a 15x10x1-in. preparing dish covered with cooking shower; sprinkle with 1-1/2 teaspoons oil. In a small bowl, blend rosemary, thyme and pepper; sprinkle half over chicken.
2. In a huge bowl, consolidate artichoke hearts, onion, wine, garlic, remaining oil and remaining spice blend; throw to cover. Orchestrate around chicken. Sprinkle chicken with cheddar; top with lemon cuts.
3. Broil until a thermometer embedded in chicken peruses 165°, 20-25 minutes. Sprinkle with green onions.

21. Sheet Pan Honey-Soy Salmon

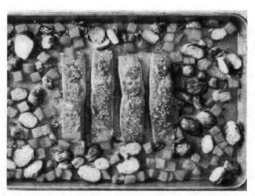

Active Time: 15 Mins | Total Time: 42 Mins | Yield: Serves 4 (1 salmon fillet, about 2/3 cup squash, and 2/3 cup Brussels sprouts)

Ingredients

- Cooking splash
- 1/2 tablespoon lower-sodium soy sauce or tamari
- 3 tablespoons olive oil, separated
- 1 tablespoon nectar
- 1 tablespoon new lime juice (from 1 lime)
- 2 cloves garlic, minced, partitioned
- 1/2 teaspoon newly ground ginger
- 4 (5 oz.) skin-on salmon filets
- 2 1/2 cups butternut squash, stripped and cubed
- 12 ounces Brussels grows, managed and split
- 1/2 teaspoon legitimate salt
- 1/2 teaspoon newly ground dark pepper
- 1/4 teaspoon smoked paprika
- 1 tablespoon cut green onion

- 1 teaspoon sesame seeds

DIRECTION:
1. Preheat oven to 400°F. Coat a 13 x 18-inch half sheet dish with cooking splash.
2. Consolidate soy sauce, 1 tablespoon of the oil, nectar, lime juice, 1 clove of garlic, and ginger in an enormous bowl. Spot salmon in bowl. Throw to cover. Put in a safe spot.
3. In a different bowl, consolidate remaining 2 tablespoons of oil, remaining clove of garlic, butternut squash, Brussels sprouts, salt, pepper, and paprika. Throw to cover. Spread on preparing sheet, abstaining from congestion. Heat at 400°F for 12 minutes. Mix vegetables and push to edges of skillet, making an open place.
4. Spot marinated salmon filets in the open community space of container. Pour any extra marinade over salmon. Prepare at 400° for 15 minutes. Top salmon with green onion and sesame seeds. Present with squash and Brussels sprouts.

22. Beef Salad

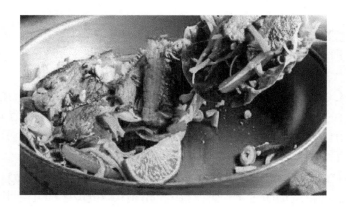

Prep Time: 20 mins | Cook Time: 20 mins | Total Time: 40 mins | Servings: 4 servings Calories: 384kcal

Ingredients

- Marinated Beef
- 320 g sirloin steak (approx. 2 steaks – fat eliminated)
- 2 tbsp. clam sauce
- 1 tsp. dim soy sauce
- 1 tbsp. corn flour
- 1 tbsp. sunflower oil
- Crunchy Slaw
- 400 g white cabbage (meagerly destroyed)
- 160 g mange promote (finely cut)
- 1 medium carrot (cut into fine cudgel)
- 1 red onion (finely cut)
- 1 red pepper (finely cut)
- Slaw Dressing
- 2 tbsp. sunflower oil
- 1 tbsp. light soy sauce

- 4 tbsp. rice wine vinegar (can substitute with red wine vinegar)
- 2 tbsp. lime juice
- 2 tsp. sesame oil
- 1 clove garlic squashed
- 1 red bean stew (de-cultivated and finely cut)
- 1 tbsp. root ginger (finely ground)
- 1 tbsp. mint leaves (finely destroyed)
- To Serve
- 2 little jewel lettuce (forgets about isolated)
- 4 spring onions (finely cut)
- 4 tbsp. peanuts (squashed)
- 1 lime (cut into wedges)
- 1 little bundle new mint leaves

Instructions:

1. Marinated Beef
2. Spot the clam sauce, dim soy sauce and corn flour into a bowl and blend well to join to a smooth paste. Add the entire sirloin steaks to the marinade and blend to guarantee the steaks are totally covered. Put in a safe spot for 15 minutes while you set up the remainder of the dish.
3. Asian Slaw
4. Set up every one of the vegetables for the Asian slaw and spot them in an enormous bowl. Put in a safe spot.
5. In a bowl combine as one every one of the ingredients for the slaw dressing and mix well to join. Pour over the vegetables and blend completely through the vegetables. Put to the side until prepared to serve.
6. To serve

7. At the point when prepared to serve, place a huge non-stick griddle over a high heat. Add 1tbsp sunflower oil to the griddle and spot the steaks into the skillet to cook for 2-3 minutes on each side.
8. The timeframe will change contingent upon the thickness of the steaks. However, for a medium cooked steak you are searching for an interior temperature of 60-65C.
9. At the point when the steak is cooked, eliminate from the container and put to the side on a warm plate to rest for 5 minutes.
10. In the interim set up the lettuce leaves and spot a spoon of the slaw into every one of the leaves.
11. When rested cut every sirloin steak into slender cuts and a few cuts onto every lettuce leaf. Trimming with spring onion, squashed peanuts, new torn mint leaves and a wedge of new lime. Serve right away.
12. On the off chance that you don't care for bean stew avoid it with regards to the dressing completely.
13. The trimming things are a serving idea in particular. In the event that you have a nut hypersensitivity leaves the nuts off the dish.

23. Tacos with Lime-Cilantro Cremal

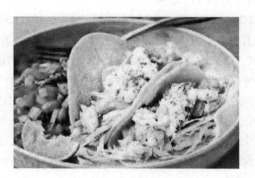

Total: 15 mins | Yield: 4 servings (serving size: 2 tacos)

Ingredients

- Crema:
- ¼ cup daintily cut green onions
- ¼ cup chopped new cilantro
- 3 tablespoons without fat mayonnaise
- 3 tablespoons decreased fat sharp cream
- 1 teaspoon ground lime skin
- 1 ½ teaspoons new lime juice
- ¼ teaspoon salt
- 1 garlic clove, minced
- Tacos:
- 1 teaspoon ground cumin
- 1 teaspoon ground coriander
- ½ teaspoon smoked paprika
- ¼ teaspoon ground red pepper
- ⅛ teaspoon salt
- ⅛ teaspoon garlic powder
- 1 ½ pounds red snapper filets
- Cooking shower

- 8 (6-inch) corn tortillas
- 2 cups shredded cabbage

Directions

1. Preheat oven to 425°.
2. To plan crema, consolidate the initial 8 ingredients in a little bowl; put in a safe spot.
3. To get ready tacos, consolidate cumin and next 5 ingredients (through garlic powder) in a little bowl; sprinkle zest combination uniformly over the two sides of fish. Spot fish on a heating sheet covered with cooking shower. Prepare at 425° for 9 minutes or until fish chips effectively when tried with a fork or until wanted level of doneness. Spot fish in a bowl; break into pieces with a fork. Heat tortillas as per bundle directions. Separation fish uniformly among tortillas; top each with 1/4 cup cabbage and 1 tablespoon cremal.

24. Vegetable & Lentil Salad

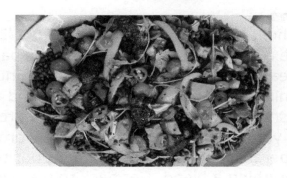

Prep Time 10 minutes | Cook Time 45 minutes | Total Time 55 minutes | Servings 2 people

INGREDIENTS

- 2 little yams stripped and cut into 1 inch shapes
- 100 g (1/2 pack) chestnut mushrooms quartered
- 10 cherry/plum tomatoes
- 1 yellow pepper cut into 1/2 inch strips
- 1/2 head broccoli cut into florets
- 1/2 tbsp. olive oil
- 1 tsp. stew chips
- Ocean salt and newly ground dark pepper
- 100 g (1/2 cup) dry puy lentils/lentilles vertes
- **FOR THE DRESSING**
- 15 g (1/2 pack) new coriander
- 2 tbsp. common yogurt
- 1 clove garlic stripped
- Juice of 1/2 a lemon
- Touch of ocean salt
- **TO SERVE**

- 60 g (1 sack) wild rocket
- 15 g (1/2 pack) coriander leaves as it were
- 1 red stew meagerly cut

Directions

1. Preheat the oven to 170°c fan/190°c/375°f.
2. Line a preparing plate with material paper and spread over the yam. Cook for 10 minutes.
3. Eliminate the plate from the oven and add the mushrooms, tomatoes, pepper and broccoli to the yam. Shower over the oil, stew drops and a liberal spot of salt and pepper prior to giving everything a blend. Get back to the oven for another 30-35 minutes until the vegetables are delicate and cooked through.
4. Then spot the lentils in a medium sauce container and cover with cold water. Carry the container to bubble prior to decreasing the heat and stewing delicately for 18-20 minutes until delicate. Channel and put in a safe spot.
5. To make the dressing place the coriander, yogurt, garlic, lemon squeeze and salt into a blender/food processor. Mix until smooth. Taste and change the flavoring if necessary.
6. To gather, blend the rocket, lentils and 2/3rds of the broiled vegetables together in an enormous bowl. Move onto a serving platter and top with the leftover simmered veg, coriander and stew cuts. Generously shower over the dressing and serve!
7. Formula NOTES
8. This serving of mixed greens can be enjoyed hot or cold! To serve cold simply permit every one of the components to cool totally prior to

gathering and putting away in the ice chest. Add the dressing not long prior to serving.

9. This serving of mixed greens is ideal for lunch boxes as it saves truly well for an as long as 4 days in the cooler. I like to make a twofold bunch of this cooked vegetable and lentil serving of mixed greens toward the start of the week to save for a fast and sound lunch.

10. You can switch up the vegetables in this serving of mixed greens to whatever you have at home/what is in season. I love this with courgette and aubergine as well - simply recall that cooking times will shift!!

11. For this lentil serving of mixed greens I use puy lentils/lentilles vertes (not to be mistaken for green lentils) which you can without much of a stretch find in any grocery store. In the event that you are feeling sluggish you can likewise utilize 250g of pre-cooked lentils - I here and there utilize these ones!

12. To make this plate of mixed greens veggie lover simply trade the yogurt for a dairy free option, for example, soya yogurt in the dressing.

25. Roasted Butternut Squash Cauliflower Salad

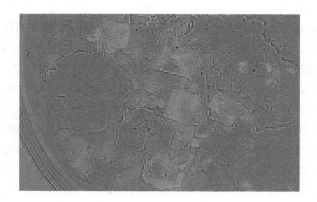

SERVINGS: 4 PEOPLE | PREP TIME: 10 MINUTES | COOK TIME: 20 MINUTES | TOTAL TIME: 30 MINUTES

Ingredients
FOR THE SALAD

- 1 medium cauliflower head - cut into florets
- 1 little butternut squash - stripped and cut in 3D squares
- 1 tbsp. olive oil
- salt and dark pepper
- ¼ cup red onion - chopped
- 1 tablespoon green onions - chopped
- **FOR DRESSING**
- 1/2 cup vegenaise or customary mayonnaise
- 2 tablespoon yellow mustard
- 1 teaspoon garlic - minced
- Salt and pepper

Guidelines

1. To begin with, steam the head of cauliflower. In an enormous pot add around 2 cups of water and spot a liner crate in the base.
2. Heat the water to the point of boiling. Add the cauliflower florets into the liner crate.
3. Cover the pot and steam until the cauliflower florets are delicate 6-8 minutes. The time will rely upon how delicate you incline toward your cauliflower florets to be.
4. Eliminate from the heat and furthermore eliminate the top from the pot. Allow the cauliflower to chill off for 5 minutes.
5. While the cauliflower florets are been steamed, cook the butternut squash. Preheat oven to 400 degrees. On a heating sheet fixed with material paper or silicone tangle, place butternut squash and throw in olive oil and season with salt and dark pepper. Blend well to consolidate.
6. Cook in the oven for 15-20 minutes (It'll rely upon the size of the butternut squash diced).
7. Spot the steamed cauliflower, the simmered butternut squash and the red onions in a bowl.
8. In a little glass bowl, add every one of the ingredients for the dressing and whisk all that together to consolidate.
9. Taste to check the flavoring and pour over the serving of mixed greens.
10. Combine every one of the ingredients as one until very much consolidated and trimming it with green onions.

26. Easy seafood soup

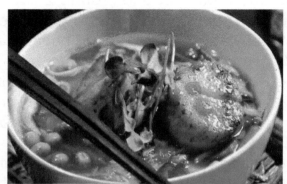

22 MINUTES | SERVINGS: 2 BOWLS

INGREDIENTS
- 2½ C vegetable stock
- 4 ocean scallops, washed and wiped off
- 2 C gluten free noodles, cooked as coordinated
- 1 carrot, stripped and julienned
- 2 celery ribs, meagerly cut
- 2 red radish, managed and daintily cut
- 1 C spring peas, shelled, pods disposed of
- 2 C shiitake mushroom covers, daintily cut
- 1 scallion, managed and daintily cut
- 2 cloves garlic, shredded
- 1 T new ginger, cleaned and shredded
- 1 T unsalted spread
- 1 T additional virgin olive oil
- 1 tsp. fit salt, more to taste
- run sriracha or other hot sauce
- embellish with sprinkling of miniature greens

DIRECTIONS

1. Wash and afterward strip, trim, cut hack, cut, dice or julienne vegetables as you wish. Wash ocean scallops and afterward wipe off.
2. Empty vegetable stock into a medium-sized pot. Heat to the point of boiling and afterward decrease to stew. Mix in garlic, ginger and salt. Cover.
3. Heat 5 cups of salted water to the point of boiling. Add dried noodles and cook as coordinated. Channel and gap into two soup bowls.
4. Simultaneously, carry a medium measured skillet to medium-high temperature. Add spread and olive oil, permitting them to mix and come to temperature. Add scallops, being mindful so as not to swarm them in the skillet. Burn one side, around 3-4 minutes, turn over and rehash. When cooked, eliminate from skillet and permit to rest.
5. Return stock to a bubble. Add vegetables and cook for 4 minutes.
6. Using an opened spoon, eliminate the entirety of the vegetables from the stock. Spoon onto cooked noodles, partitioning them uniformly between the two dishes.
7. Move two singed scallops into each bowl. Spoon equivalent measures of bubbling stock into each bowl.
8. Add a scramble of hot sauce to each bowl and trimming both with a sprinkling of micro greens.

27. Salmon And Vegetables

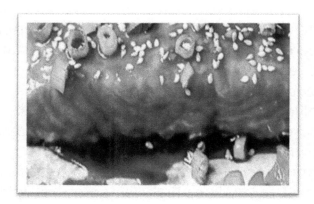

Prep time: 15 mins | cook time: 20 mins | total time: 35 mins

INGREDIENTS

- **For vegetables:**
- 2 cups reduced down broccoli florets
- 10 scaled down sweet rainbow peppers, cultivated and divided
- 1 tablespoon sesame oil
- ¼ teaspoon genuine salt
- Newly ground dark pepper, to taste
- **For salmon:**
- 2 (4-ounce) wild salmon filets
- 1 teaspoon sesame oil
- 1 garlic clove, ground
- ½ teaspoon ground ginger
- 2 tablespoons diminished sodium soy sauce, or sans gluten soy sauce
- 1 teaspoon unseasoned rice vinegar
- 1 teaspoon brown sugar

- **For decorate:**
- ½ teaspoon toasted sesame seeds
- 1 enormous scallion, chopped

Instructions:

1. Preheat oven to 400F degrees. Cover an enormous sheet skillet with foil or material, gently shower olive oil and put in a safe spot.
2. In the mean time, join sesame oil, garlic, ginger, soy sauce, vinegar and brown sugar in a little bowl and blend. Fill a huge zip lock sack and add salmon, marinate 10 minutes.
3. salmon in marinade
4. In a medium bowl, throw broccoli and peppers with 1 tablespoon sesame oil, ¼ teaspoon salt and pepper. Spread them uniformly on arranged sheet container and meal for 10 minutes.
5. Eliminate veggies from oven, throw, and move them over somewhat to account for the salmon. Spot the salmon on the sheet skillet, holding the marinade and get back to oven, broil an extra 7 to 8 minutes, or until salmon is simply cooked through.
6. While salmon is cooking, heat a little skillet over low heat. Pour the leftover marinade and stew mixing until the sauce has thickened somewhat, around 1 to 1/2 minutes.
7. Brush sauce over salmon and sprinkle filets with sesame seeds and scallions. Present with veggies as an afterthought

28. Lemon Chicken Ozrp Soup

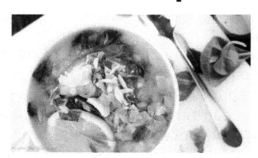

INGREDIENTS
- 2-tablespoons of olive oil, divided
- 1-boneless pound, some thighs, cut into 1-chunks
- Kosher salt and freshly ground black pepper
- 3-cloves of garlic, finely chopped
- 1-onion, diced
- 3-carrots, peeled and diced
- 2-celery stalks, cut into cubes
- 1/2 teaspoon of dried thyme
- 5 cups of chicken stock
- 2-bay leaves
- 3/4 cup uncooked orzo pasta
- 1-sprig of rosemary
- Juice of 1 lemon
- 2-tablespoons of chopped fresh parsley leaves

DIRECTIONS
1. Heat 1-tablespoon of olive oil in a large stockpot or Dutch oven over medium heat. Season chicken thighs with salt and pepper to taste. Add chook to the stockpot and cook dinner until golden brown, about 2-3 minutes; put aside.

2. Add the remaining 1-tablespoon of oil to the stockpot. Add garlic, onion, carrots, and celery. Cook, occasionally stirring, until tender, about three to four minutes. Stay in thyme until fragrant, about 1 minute.
3. Beat in bird inventory, bay leaves, and 1 cup of water; bring to a boil. Stir in orzo, rosemary, and chicken; reduce heat and simmer until orzo is cooked for about 10-12 minutes.

29. Super Food Paleo Soup

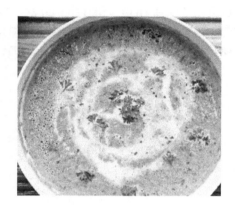

***Hands-on 10 minutes Overall 20 minute|
serving size about 1 1/2 cups/ 360 ml***

INGREDIENTS:

- 1 medium head cauliflower (400 g/14.1 oz.)
- 1 medium white onion (110 g/3.9 oz.)
- 2 cloves garlic
- 1 straight leaf, disintegrated
- 150 g watercress (5.3 oz.)
- 200 g new spinach (7.1 oz.) or frozen spinach (220 g/7.8 oz.)
- 1 liter vegetable stock or bone stock or chicken stock (4 cups/1 quart) - you can make your own
- 1 cup cream or coconut milk (240 ml/8 fl. oz.) + 6 tbsp. for decorate
- 1/4 cup ghee or virgin coconut oil (55 g/1.9 oz.)

- ocean salt and ground pepper, to taste
- Discretionary: new spices like parsley or chives for embellish

Directions

1. Strip and finely dice the onion and garlic. Spot in a soup pot or a Dutch oven lubed with ghee and cook over a medium-high heat until somewhat browned. Wash the spinach and watercress and put in a safe spot.
2. Cut the cauliflower into little florets and spot in the pot with browned onion. Add disintegrated straight leaf. Cook for around 5 minutes and blend oftentimes.
3. Add the spinach and watercress and cook until shriveled for pretty many 2-3 minutes.
4. Pour in the vegetable stock and heat to the point of boiling. Cook until the cauliflower is fresh delicate and pour in the cream (or coconut milk).
5. Season with salt and pepper. Remove the heat and using a hand blender, beat until smooth and rich.
6. Serve promptly or chill and keep refrigerated for as long as 5 days. Freeze for longer. Just prior to serving, sprinkle some cream on top. Store in the refrigerator for as long as 5 days or freeze for as long as 3 months.

30. Chicken with Broccoli and Sweet Potato Wedges

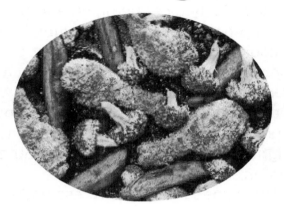

Prep time: 30 min | Serves 4

Ingredients

- 8 (3 1/2-oz.) chicken drumsticks, cleaned
- 1 tablespoon new lemon juice
- 1/8 teaspoons kosher salt, isolated
- 1/2 teaspoon poultry preparing
- 1 teaspoon garlic powder, separated
- 1/8 teaspoon newly ground dark pepper
- 2 huge eggs, gently thumped
- 1 cup panko (Japanese breadcrumbs)
- 1/2 ounces Parmesan cheddar, ground (around 1/3 cup)
- 1 teaspoon dried oregano
- 1 teaspoon dried parsley pieces (optional)
- Cooking splash 2 (7-oz.) yams, each cut into 8 wedges
- 2 tablespoons olive oil, partitioned
- 1/2 teaspoon paprika
- 1/2 teaspoon bean stew powder

- 7 cups broccoli florets (around 12 oz.)
- 1 garlic clove, squashed or ground 5 lemon wedges

Directions:
1. Preheat oven to 425°F.
2. Spot chicken in an enormous bowl. Shower with lemon squeeze, and sprinkle with 3/8 teaspoon salt, poultry preparing, 1/2 teaspoon garlic powder, and dark pepper; throw to join.
3. Spot eggs in a shallow dish. Consolidate panko, Parmesan, oregano, and parsley, if using, in another shallow dish. Plunge every drumstick in eggs at that point dig in panko blend. Spot drumsticks on a rimmed heating sheet covered with cooking shower; dispose of outstanding egg and panko blend. Coat highest points of drumsticks with cooking splash. Prepare at 425°F for 15 minutes.
4. Consolidate potatoes, 1 tablespoon oil, staying 1/2 teaspoon garlic powder, paprika, bean stew powder, and 3/8 teaspoon salt; throw to cover. Mastermind potatoes on one portion of another rimmed preparing sheet covered with cooking shower. Spot in oven with chicken, and heat at 425°F for 10 minutes.
5. Consolidate broccoli, staying 1 tablespoon oil, garlic clove, and staying 3/8 teaspoon salt. Eliminate heating sheet with potatoes from oven; turn potatoes over, and add broccoli to other portion of container. Spot in oven with chicken, and heat at 425°F for 20 minutes or until chicken and potatoes are finished. Crush

1 lemon wedge over broccoli. Serve remaining lemon wedges with the dinner.

31. Corn Quinoa Salad

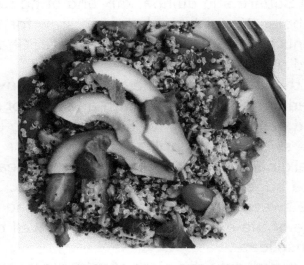

Prep Time 10 minutes| Cook Time 15 minutes|
Total Time 25 minutes| Servings 2 servings

INGREDIENTS

- 100 g (2/3 cup) quinoa washed
- 1/4 vegetable stock 3D square
- 1 tsp. rapeseed/olive oil
- 200 g tin of sweet corn depleted
- 100 g (huge small bunch) cherry/plum tomatoes quartered
- 1 huge small bunch coriander generally chopped
- 4 spring onions finely cut
- Squeeze and zing of 1 lime
- 1/2 tsp. stew chips
- 1 ready avocado stripped and cut
- Liberal squeeze ocean salt and newly ground dark pepper

Directions

1. Fill a medium pot with water and add the stock 3D Square and quinoa, mix and bring to the bubble. Diminish the heat and stew for 15-18 minutes until the quinoa is delicate. Channel and put in a safe spot.

2. In the interim, heat the oil in a skillet over a medium heat. Add the corn and spot of salt and pepper and fry for 5 minutes or so until the sweet corn is brilliant brown and marginally fresh. Eliminate from the heat.

3. In a huge bowl add the cooked quinoa, 3/4 of the sweet corn, 3/4 of the avocado and every one of the excess ingredients. Mix well to consolidate.

4. To serve, split the plate of mixed greens between two plates prior to embellishing with the excess sweet corn and avocado.

5. Formula NOTES

6. This serving of mixed greens is extraordinary hot or cold! To serve cold permit both the quinoa and sweet corn to totally cool. At that point consolidate with the leftover ingredients and refrigerate.

7. In the event that you plan to pre-make this Mexican toasted corn quinoa plate of mixed greens, overlook the avocado (so it doesn't brown), keep the pre-made serving of mixed greens in a water/air proof holder in the cooler for as long as 3 days and add the avocado not long prior to serving.

8. Ensure that your tinned sweet corn hasn't got any additional sugar or salt. The ingredients

should peruse 'sweet corn, water' as it were. It is smarter to add the salt yourself!

9. In my formula I have utilized a tri-shading quinoa (white, red and dark). However, white quinoa will function admirably!

10.   Watch out for undesirable ingredients on your stock 3D squares. I utilize the Kallo exceptionally low salt stock solid shapes - they are incredible!

32. Glazed Salmon with Veggies and Oranges

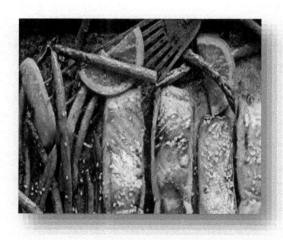

***Hands-On: 25 mins | total: 25 mins| Yield:
Makes 4 servings***

Ingredients
- 4 tablespoons nectar
- 1 tablespoon soy sauce
- 1 tablespoon Dijon mustard
- 1 teaspoon prepared rice wine vinegar
- ¼ teaspoon dried squashed red pepper
- 1 pound new medium asparagus
- 8 ounces new green beans, managed
- 1 little orange, cut into 1/4-to 1/2-inch cuts
- 1 tablespoon olive oil
- 1 teaspoon legitimate salt
- ¼ teaspoon newly ground dark pepper
- 4 (5-to 6-oz.) new salmon filets

- Topping: toasted sesame seeds

Directions

1. Preheat oven with oven rack 6 crawls from heat. Whisk together nectar and next 4 ingredients in a little bowl.
2. Snap off and dispose of intense closures of asparagus. Spot asparagus, green beans, and next 4 ingredients in an enormous bowl, and throw to cover.
3. Spot salmon in focus of a substantial aluminum foil-lined sheet container. Brush salmon with around 2 Tbsp. nectar combinations. Spread asparagus combination around salmon.
4. Cook 4 minutes; eliminate from oven, and brush salmon with around 2 Tbsp. nectar combination. Get back to oven, and sear 4 minutes more. Eliminate from oven, and brush salmon with remaining nectar blend. Get back to oven, and cook 2 minutes more. Serve right away.

33. Turkey and Peppers

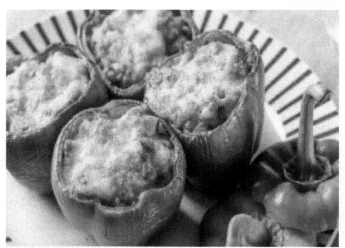

INGREDIENTS:

- 1 teaspoon of salt, divided
- 1 pound turkey fillet, cut into thin steaks of about ¼ inch thick sliced
- 2 tablespoons of extra virgin olive oil, divided
- ½ large sweet onion, sliced
- 1 red pepper, cut into strips
- 1 yellow pepper, cut into strips
- ½ teaspoon of Italian herbs
- ¼ teaspoon ground black pepper
- 2 teaspoons of red wine vinegar
- 1 14-ounce tomato, preferably fire-roasted
- Chopped fresh parsley and basil for garnish (optional)

DIRECTIONS:

1. Sprinkle ½ teaspoon of salt over turkey—heat 1 tablespoon of oil in a large non-stick frying pan over medium heat. Add half of the turkey and cook until brown on the bottom, 1 to 3 minutes. Flip and continue to cook until completely cooked 1 to 2 minutes. Place the turkey on a plate with a slotted spatula, tent with foil to keep warm. Add the remaining 1 tablespoon of oil to the pan, reduce the heat to medium and repeat with the remaining turkey, 1 to 3 minutes per side.

2. Add onion, bell pepper, and remaining ½ teaspoon of salt to the pan, cover, and cook, removing the lid to stir often until onion and bell pepper turn soft and blotchy brown, 5 to 7 minutes. Remove lid, increase heat to medium-low, drizzle with Italian herbs and pepper, and cook, often stirring, until spices are fragrant, about 30 seconds. Add vinegar and cook, stirring until almost completely evaporated, about 20 seconds. Add tomatoes and bring to a boil, stirring frequently.

3. Add the turkey to the pan with any accumulated juices from the plate and bring it to a boil. Reduce heat to medium-low and cook, turning sauce over until turkey is completely hot, 1 to 2 minutes. Serve with parsley and basil if desired.

34. Sweet mushroom Potato Carbonara

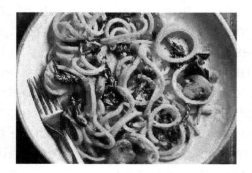

Total: 40 mins | Servings: 5 (10 plates for 50)

Ingredients

- 2 pounds yams, stripped
- 3 huge eggs, beaten
- 1 cup ground Parmesan cheese
- ¼ teaspoon salt
- ¼ teaspoon ground pepper
- 1 tablespoon extra-virgin olive oil
- 3 strips community cut bacon, chopped
- 1 8-ounce bundle cut mushrooms
- 2 cloves garlic, minced
- 1 5-ounce bundle child spinach

Directions:

1. Put a huge pot of water on to bubble.
2. Using a winding vegetable slicer or julienne vegetable peeler, cut yams longwise into long, dainty strands. You ought to have around 12 cups of "noodles."
3. Cook the yams in the bubbling water, delicately mixing on more than one occasion,

until simply beginning to mellow however not totally delicate, 1/2 to 3 minutes. Hold 1/4 cup of the cooking water, at that point channel. Return the noodles to the pot, off the heat. Consolidate eggs, Parmesan, salt, pepper and the held water in a bowl; pour over the noodles and tenderly throw with utensils until uniformly covered.

4. Heat oil in a huge skillet over medium heat. Add bacon and mushrooms and cook, mixing regularly, until the fluid has dissipated and the mushrooms are beginning to brown, 6 to 8 minutes. Add garlic and cook, blending, until fragrant, around 1 moment. Add spinach and cook, mixing, until shriveled, 1 to 2 minutes. Add the vegetables to the noodles and throw to join. Top with a liberal pounding of pepper.

35. Fried eggs in spiced yogurt

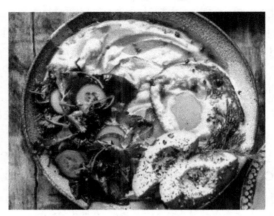

INGREDIENTS:

- 1 cup of plain Greek yogurt
- 1-tablespoon of fresh dill chopped
- 1-tablespoon fresh chopped parsley
- 2-cloves of garlic finely chopped or grated
- salt + pepper to taste
- 4-eggs
- 4-pieces of naan
- zest of 1 lemon
- 1/4 cup sun-dried tomato pesto, homemade or store-bought
- 1-2 cups of fresh baby spinach
- 4 ounces of goat cheese crumbled
- toasted sesame seeds, fresh dill, fresh mint, and salt to serve
- SPICY BUTTER SAUCE
- Two tablespoons of butter
- Two tablespoons of coconut oil
- 1-2 teaspoons ground red pepper flakes
- 1/2 teaspoon sweet paprika

DIRECTIONS:

1. In a bowl, combine the Greek yogurt, dill, parsley, garlic, and a pinch of salt + pepper. Stir until combined. Keep in the refrigerator until use.
2. Heat a frying pan with a little olive oil or butter over medium heat and fry the eggs as desired.
3. Divide the yogurt sauce over a piece of warm / roasted naan. Spoon 1-2 tablespoons of the sun-dried tomato pesto into the yogurt. Then add 1-2 eggs per piece. Sprinkle each piece with lemon zest and fresh spinach. Drizzle the spicy butter sauce (recipe below) over the eggs. Garnish with fresh herbs, sesame seeds, and some crumbled goat cheese. FOOD!
4. SPICY BUTTER SAUCE
5. In a small saucepan, melt with butter, coconut oil, crushed red pepper flakes, and paprika. Drizzle the warm sauce over the fried eggs.

Conclusion

I would like to thank you for picking this book. This includes recipes for diabetic patients which are easy to prepare at home and are very rich in nutrients. These recipes can be easily prepared within less time. Try at home and appreciate.

I wish you all good luck!

Lightning Source UK Ltd.
Milton Keynes UK
UKHW020701240521
384264UK00005B/52